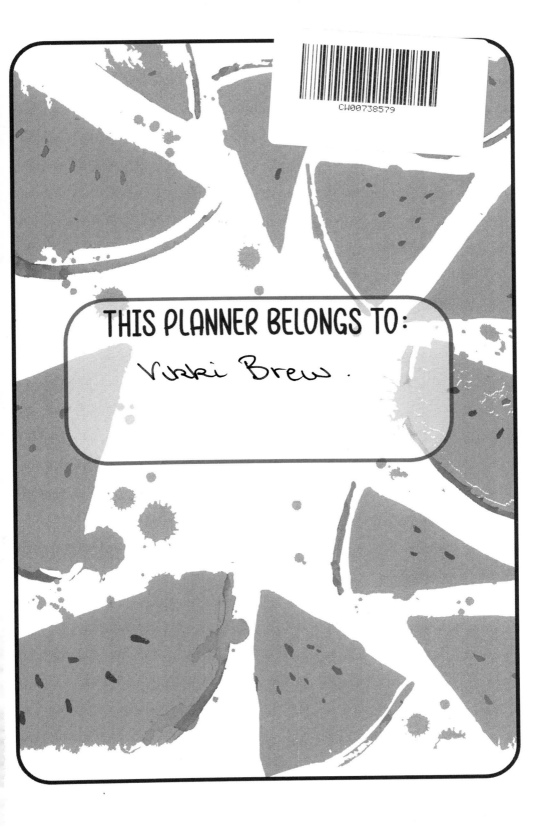

THIS PLANNER BELONGS TO:

Vikki Brew .

Cooking with love provides food for the soul

MEAL PLANNER

DATE:

	BREAKFAST	LUNCH	DINNER
MONDAY		Salad	Frikadelin + roast veg
TUESDAY			
WEDNESDAY			
THURSDAY			
FRIDAY			
SATURDAY	Oat Flakes + milk	1x cheese + onion crisps	Cheese on toast
SUNDAY	2x Weetabix milk	fruit salad	Aubergine Stir fry.

Delicious!

MONDAY

SNACKS

TUESDAY

SNACKS

WEDNESDAY

SNACKS

THURSDAY

SNACKS

FRIDAY

SNACKS

SATURDAY

SNACKS

1 mint twirl.
2x malted milk

SUNDAY

SNACKS

GROCERY LIST

- yoghurts
- mozzerela
- parmasen substitute
-
- Celerac
- Swede
- Cauli.
- pots.
-
- milk   etc.

NOTES:

MEAL PLANNER

pinch of nom
1st book.

DATE:

	BREAKFAST	LUNCH	DINNER
MONDAY	weetabix	Salad Tuna.	Veg biriyani pge 62
TUESDAY			Spiced salmon pge 94
WEDNESDAY			Chicken + leeks in blue cheese pge 112.
THURSDAY			DINNER Pge ~~goulash~~ 168. ~~pge two~~ Pork + lentils
FRIDAY			goulash Pge 140 ~~Pork on balsamic lentils.~~
SATURDAY			(BBQ)
SUNDAY			(Chicken roast)

Tasty!

MONDAY
SNACKS

TUESDAY
SNACKS

WEDNESDAY
SNACKS

THURSDAY
SNACKS

FRIDAY
SNACKS

SATURDAY
SNACKS

SUNDAY
SNACKS

GROCERY LIST

- _____
- _____
- _____
- _____
- _____
- _____
- _____
- _____
- _____
- _____
- _____
- _____
- _____
- _____
- _____
- _____
- _____
- _____
- _____
- _____
- _____
- _____
- _____
- _____

NOTES:

MEAL PLANNER

DATE:

	BREAKFAST	LUNCH	DINNER
MONDAY			

	BREAKFAST	LUNCH	DINNER
TUESDAY			

	BREAKFAST	LUNCH	DINNER
WEDNESDAY			

	BREAKFAST	LUNCH	DINNER
THURSDAY			

	BREAKFAST	LUNCH	DINNER
FRIDAY			

	BREAKFAST	LUNCH	DINNER
SATURDAY			

	BREAKFAST	LUNCH	DINNER
SUNDAY			

scrumptious!

GROCERY LIST

MONDAY SNACKS

TUESDAY SNACKS

WEDNESDAY SNACKS

THURSDAY SNACKS

FRIDAY SNACKS

SATURDAY SNACKS

SUNDAY SNACKS

NOTES:

MEAL PLANNER

DATE:

MONDAY
BREAKFAST	LUNCH	DINNER

TUESDAY
BREAKFAST	LUNCH	DINNER

WEDNESDAY
BREAKFAST	LUNCH	DINNER

THURSDAY
BREAKFAST	LUNCH	DINNER

FRIDAY
BREAKFAST	LUNCH	DINNER

SATURDAY
BREAKFAST	LUNCH	DINNER

SUNDAY
BREAKFAST	LUNCH	DINNER

Delectable!

GROCERY LIST

MONDAY
SNACKS

TUESDAY
SNACKS

WEDNESDAY
SNACKS

THURSDAY
SNACKS

FRIDAY
SNACKS

SATURDAY
SNACKS

SUNDAY
SNACKS

NOTES:

MEAL PLANNER

DATE:

MONDAY	BREAKFAST	LUNCH	DINNER

TUESDAY	BREAKFAST	LUNCH	DINNER

WEDNESDAY	BREAKFAST	LUNCH	DINNER

THURSDAY	BREAKFAST	LUNCH	DINNER

FRIDAY	BREAKFAST	LUNCH	DINNER

SATURDAY	BREAKFAST	LUNCH	DINNER

SUNDAY	BREAKFAST	LUNCH	DINNER

yummy!

MONDAY
SNACKS

TUESDAY
SNACKS

WEDNESDAY
SNACKS

THURSDAY
SNACKS

FRIDAY
SNACKS

SATURDAY
SNACKS

SUNDAY
SNACKS

GROCERY LIST

- _____
- _____
- _____
- _____
- _____
- _____
- _____
- _____
- _____
- _____
- _____
- _____
- _____
- _____
- _____
- _____
- _____
- _____
- _____
- _____
- _____

NOTES:

MEAL PLANNER

DATE:

MONDAY
BREAKFAST	LUNCH	DINNER

TUESDAY
BREAKFAST	LUNCH	DINNER

WEDNESDAY
BREAKFAST	LUNCH	DINNER

THURSDAY
BREAKFAST	LUNCH	DINNER

FRIDAY
BREAKFAST	LUNCH	DINNER

SATURDAY
BREAKFAST	LUNCH	DINNER

SUNDAY
BREAKFAST	LUNCH	DINNER

Delicious!

MONDAY
SNACKS

TUESDAY
SNACKS

WEDNESDAY
SNACKS

THURSDAY
SNACKS

FRIDAY
SNACKS

SATURDAY
SNACKS

SUNDAY
SNACKS

GROCERY LIST

- _____
- _____
- _____
- _____
- _____
- _____
- _____
- _____
- _____
- _____
- _____
- _____
- _____
- _____
- _____
- _____
- _____
- _____
- _____
- _____
- _____
- _____
- _____

NOTES:

MEAL PLANNER

DATE:

	BREAKFAST	LUNCH	DINNER
MONDAY			

	BREAKFAST	LUNCH	DINNER
TUESDAY			

	BREAKFAST	LUNCH	DINNER
WEDNESDAY			

	BREAKFAST	LUNCH	DINNER
THURSDAY			

	BREAKFAST	LUNCH	DINNER
FRIDAY			

	BREAKFAST	LUNCH	DINNER
SATURDAY			

	BREAKFAST	LUNCH	DINNER
SUNDAY			

Tasty!

MONDAY
SNACKS

TUESDAY
SNACKS

WEDNESDAY
SNACKS

THURSDAY
SNACKS

FRIDAY
SNACKS

SATURDAY
SNACKS

SUNDAY
SNACKS

GROCERY LIST

- _____
- _____
- _____
- _____
- _____
- _____
- _____
- _____
- _____
- _____
- _____
- _____
- _____
- _____
- _____
- _____
- _____
- _____
- _____
- _____
- _____
- _____

NOTES:

MEAL PLANNER

DATE:

MONDAY	BREAKFAST	LUNCH	DINNER

TUESDAY	BREAKFAST	LUNCH	DINNER

WEDNESDAY	BREAKFAST	LUNCH	DINNER

THURSDAY	BREAKFAST	LUNCH	DINNER

FRIDAY	BREAKFAST	LUNCH	DINNER

SATURDAY	BREAKFAST	LUNCH	DINNER

SUNDAY	BREAKFAST	LUNCH	DINNER

scrumptious!

GROCERY LIST

MONDAY — SNACKS

TUESDAY — SNACKS

WEDNESDAY — SNACKS

THURSDAY — SNACKS

FRIDAY — SNACKS

SATURDAY — SNACKS

SUNDAY — SNACKS

NOTES:

MEAL PLANNER

DATE:

MONDAY
BREAKFAST | LUNCH | DINNER

TUESDAY
BREAKFAST | LUNCH | DINNER

WEDNESDAY
BREAKFAST | LUNCH | DINNER

THURSDAY
BREAKFAST | LUNCH | DINNER

FRIDAY
BREAKFAST | LUNCH | DINNER

SATURDAY
BREAKFAST | LUNCH | DINNER

SUNDAY
BREAKFAST | LUNCH | DINNER

Delectable!

GROCERY LIST

MONDAY
SNACKS

TUESDAY
SNACKS

WEDNESDAY
SNACKS

THURSDAY
SNACKS

FRIDAY
SNACKS

SATURDAY
SNACKS

SUNDAY
SNACKS

NOTES:

MEAL PLANNER

DATE:

MONDAY	BREAKFAST	LUNCH	DINNER

TUESDAY	BREAKFAST	LUNCH	DINNER

WEDNESDAY	BREAKFAST	LUNCH	DINNER

THURSDAY	BREAKFAST	LUNCH	DINNER

FRIDAY	BREAKFAST	LUNCH	DINNER

SATURDAY	BREAKFAST	LUNCH	DINNER

SUNDAY	BREAKFAST	LUNCH	DINNER

yummy!

MONDAY
SNACKS

TUESDAY
SNACKS

WEDNESDAY
SNACKS

THURSDAY
SNACKS

FRIDAY
SNACKS

SATURDAY
SNACKS

SUNDAY
SNACKS

GROCERY LIST

- _____
- _____
- _____
- _____
- _____
- _____
- _____
- _____
- _____
- _____
- _____
- _____
- _____
- _____
- _____
- _____
- _____
- _____
- _____
- _____
- _____
- _____

NOTES:

MEAL PLANNER

DATE:

MONDAY	BREAKFAST	LUNCH	DINNER

TUESDAY	BREAKFAST	LUNCH	DINNER

WEDNESDAY	BREAKFAST	LUNCH	DINNER

THURSDAY	BREAKFAST	LUNCH	DINNER

FRIDAY	BREAKFAST	LUNCH	DINNER

SATURDAY	BREAKFAST	LUNCH	DINNER

SUNDAY	BREAKFAST	LUNCH	DINNER

Delicious!

MONDAY
SNACKS

TUESDAY
SNACKS

WEDNESDAY
SNACKS

THURSDAY
SNACKS

FRIDAY
SNACKS

SATURDAY
SNACKS

SUNDAY
SNACKS

GROCERY LIST

- _____
- _____
- _____
- _____
- _____
- _____
- _____
- _____
- _____
- _____
- _____
- _____
- _____
- _____
- _____
- _____
- _____
- _____
- _____
- _____
- _____
- _____

NOTES:

MEAL PLANNER

DATE:

MONDAY
| BREAKFAST | LUNCH | DINNER |

TUESDAY
| BREAKFAST | LUNCH | DINNER |

WEDNESDAY
| BREAKFAST | LUNCH | DINNER |

THURSDAY
| BREAKFAST | LUNCH | DINNER |

FRIDAY
| BREAKFAST | LUNCH | DINNER |

SATURDAY
| BREAKFAST | LUNCH | DINNER |

SUNDAY
| BREAKFAST | LUNCH | DINNER |

Tasty!

GROCERY LIST

MONDAY
SNACKS

TUESDAY
SNACKS

WEDNESDAY
SNACKS

THURSDAY
SNACKS

FRIDAY
SNACKS

SATURDAY
SNACKS

SUNDAY
SNACKS

NOTES:

MEAL PLANNER

DATE:

MONDAY
BREAKFAST	LUNCH	DINNER

TUESDAY
BREAKFAST	LUNCH	DINNER

WEDNESDAY
BREAKFAST	LUNCH	DINNER

THURSDAY
BREAKFAST	LUNCH	DINNER

FRIDAY
BREAKFAST	LUNCH	DINNER

SATURDAY
BREAKFAST	LUNCH	DINNER

SUNDAY
BREAKFAST	LUNCH	DINNER

scrumptious!

GROCERY LIST

MONDAY — SNACKS

TUESDAY — SNACKS

WEDNESDAY — SNACKS

THURSDAY — SNACKS

FRIDAY — SNACKS

SATURDAY — SNACKS

SUNDAY — SNACKS

NOTES:

MEAL PLANNER

DATE:

MONDAY	BREAKFAST	LUNCH	DINNER

TUESDAY	BREAKFAST	LUNCH	DINNER

WEDNESDAY	BREAKFAST	LUNCH	DINNER

THURSDAY	BREAKFAST	LUNCH	DINNER

FRIDAY	BREAKFAST	LUNCH	DINNER

SATURDAY	BREAKFAST	LUNCH	DINNER

SUNDAY	BREAKFAST	LUNCH	DINNER

Delectable!

GROCERY LIST

SNACKS

MONDAY

SNACKS

TUESDAY

SNACKS

WEDNESDAY

SNACKS

THURSDAY

SNACKS

FRIDAY

SNACKS

SATURDAY

SNACKS

SUNDAY

NOTES:

MEAL PLANNER

DATE:

MONDAY	BREAKFAST	LUNCH	DINNER

TUESDAY	BREAKFAST	LUNCH	DINNER

WEDNESDAY	BREAKFAST	LUNCH	DINNER

THURSDAY	BREAKFAST	LUNCH	DINNER

FRIDAY	BREAKFAST	LUNCH	DINNER

SATURDAY	BREAKFAST	LUNCH	DINNER

SUNDAY	BREAKFAST	LUNCH	DINNER

yummy!

MONDAY
SNACKS

TUESDAY
SNACKS

WEDNESDAY
SNACKS

THURSDAY
SNACKS

FRIDAY
SNACKS

SATURDAY
SNACKS

SUNDAY
SNACKS

GROCERY LIST

-
-
-
-
-
-
-
-
-
-
-
-
-
-
-
-
-
-
-
-
-
-

NOTES:

MEAL PLANNER

DATE:

MONDAY
BREAKFAST LUNCH DINNER

TUESDAY
BREAKFAST LUNCH DINNER

WEDNESDAY
BREAKFAST LUNCH DINNER

THURSDAY
BREAKFAST LUNCH DINNER

FRIDAY
BREAKFAST LUNCH DINNER

SATURDAY
BREAKFAST LUNCH DINNER

SUNDAY
BREAKFAST LUNCH DINNER

Delicious!

MONDAY
SNACKS

TUESDAY
SNACKS

WEDNESDAY
SNACKS

THURSDAY
SNACKS

FRIDAY
SNACKS

SATURDAY
SNACKS

SUNDAY
SNACKS

GROCERY LIST

-
-
-
-
-
-
-
-
-
-
-
-
-
-
-
-
-
-
-
-
-

NOTES:

MEAL PLANNER

DATE:

	BREAKFAST	LUNCH	DINNER
MONDAY			

	BREAKFAST	LUNCH	DINNER
TUESDAY			

	BREAKFAST	LUNCH	DINNER
WEDNESDAY			

	BREAKFAST	LUNCH	DINNER
THURSDAY			

	BREAKFAST	LUNCH	DINNER
FRIDAY			

	BREAKFAST	LUNCH	DINNER
SATURDAY			

	BREAKFAST	LUNCH	DINNER
SUNDAY			

Tasty!

GROCERY LIST

MONDAY

SNACKS

TUESDAY

SNACKS

WEDNESDAY

SNACKS

THURSDAY

SNACKS

FRIDAY

SNACKS

SATURDAY

SNACKS

SUNDAY

SNACKS

NOTES:

MEAL PLANNER

DATE:

MONDAY
BREAKFAST	LUNCH	DINNER

TUESDAY
BREAKFAST	LUNCH	DINNER

WEDNESDAY
BREAKFAST	LUNCH	DINNER

THURSDAY
BREAKFAST	LUNCH	DINNER

FRIDAY
BREAKFAST	LUNCH	DINNER

SATURDAY
BREAKFAST	LUNCH	DINNER

SUNDAY
BREAKFAST	LUNCH	DINNER

scrumptious!

GROCERY LIST

MONDAY — SNACKS

TUESDAY — SNACKS

WEDNESDAY — SNACKS

THURSDAY — SNACKS

FRIDAY — SNACKS

SATURDAY — SNACKS

SUNDAY — SNACKS

NOTES:

MEAL PLANNER

DATE:

MONDAY	BREAKFAST	LUNCH	DINNER

TUESDAY	BREAKFAST	LUNCH	DINNER

WEDNESDAY	BREAKFAST	LUNCH	DINNER

THURSDAY	BREAKFAST	LUNCH	DINNER

FRIDAY	BREAKFAST	LUNCH	DINNER

SATURDAY	BREAKFAST	LUNCH	DINNER

SUNDAY	BREAKFAST	LUNCH	DINNER

Delectable!

MONDAY
SNACKS

TUESDAY
SNACKS

WEDNESDAY
SNACKS

THURSDAY
SNACKS

FRIDAY
SNACKS

SATURDAY
SNACKS

SUNDAY
SNACKS

GROCERY LIST

NOTES:

MEAL PLANNER

DATE:

| MONDAY | BREAKFAST | LUNCH | DINNER |

| TUESDAY | BREAKFAST | LUNCH | DINNER |

| WEDNESDAY | BREAKFAST | LUNCH | DINNER |

| THURSDAY | BREAKFAST | LUNCH | DINNER |

| FRIDAY | BREAKFAST | LUNCH | DINNER |

| SATURDAY | BREAKFAST | LUNCH | DINNER |

| SUNDAY | BREAKFAST | LUNCH | DINNER |

yummy!

GROCERY LIST

MONDAY
SNACKS

TUESDAY
SNACKS

WEDNESDAY
SNACKS

THURSDAY
SNACKS

FRIDAY
SNACKS

SATURDAY
SNACKS

SUNDAY
SNACKS

NOTES:

MEAL PLANNER

DATE:

MONDAY	BREAKFAST	LUNCH	DINNER

TUESDAY	BREAKFAST	LUNCH	DINNER

WEDNESDAY	BREAKFAST	LUNCH	DINNER

THURSDAY	BREAKFAST	LUNCH	DINNER

FRIDAY	BREAKFAST	LUNCH	DINNER

SATURDAY	BREAKFAST	LUNCH	DINNER

SUNDAY	BREAKFAST	LUNCH	DINNER

Delicious!

MONDAY
SNACKS

TUESDAY
SNACKS

WEDNESDAY
SNACKS

THURSDAY
SNACKS

FRIDAY
SNACKS

SATURDAY
SNACKS

SUNDAY
SNACKS

GROCERY LIST

-
-
-
-
-
-
-
-
-
-
-
-
-
-
-
-
-
-
-
-
-
-
-

NOTES:

MEAL PLANNER

DATE:

| MONDAY | BREAKFAST | LUNCH | DINNER |

| TUESDAY | BREAKFAST | LUNCH | DINNER |

| WEDNESDAY | BREAKFAST | LUNCH | DINNER |

| THURSDAY | BREAKFAST | LUNCH | DINNER |

| FRIDAY | BREAKFAST | LUNCH | DINNER |

| SATURDAY | BREAKFAST | LUNCH | DINNER |

| SUNDAY | BREAKFAST | LUNCH | DINNER |

Tasty!

MONDAY
SNACKS

TUESDAY
SNACKS

WEDNESDAY
SNACKS

THURSDAY
SNACKS

FRIDAY
SNACKS

SATURDAY
SNACKS

SUNDAY
SNACKS

GROCERY LIST

-
-
-
-
-
-
-
-
-
-
-
-
-
-
-
-
-
-
-
-
-
-
-

NOTES:

MEAL PLANNER

DATE:

MONDAY	BREAKFAST	LUNCH	DINNER

TUESDAY	BREAKFAST	LUNCH	DINNER

WEDNESDAY	BREAKFAST	LUNCH	DINNER

THURSDAY	BREAKFAST	LUNCH	DINNER

FRIDAY	BREAKFAST	LUNCH	DINNER

SATURDAY	BREAKFAST	LUNCH	DINNER

SUNDAY	BREAKFAST	LUNCH	DINNER

scrumptious!

GROCERY LIST

MONDAY — SNACKS

TUESDAY — SNACKS

WEDNESDAY — SNACKS

THURSDAY — SNACKS

FRIDAY — SNACKS

SATURDAY — SNACKS

SUNDAY — SNACKS

NOTES:

MEAL PLANNER

DATE:

MONDAY
BREAKFAST	LUNCH	DINNER

TUESDAY
BREAKFAST	LUNCH	DINNER

WEDNESDAY
BREAKFAST	LUNCH	DINNER

THURSDAY
BREAKFAST	LUNCH	DINNER

FRIDAY
BREAKFAST	LUNCH	DINNER

SATURDAY
BREAKFAST	LUNCH	DINNER

SUNDAY
BREAKFAST	LUNCH	DINNER

Delectable!

GROCERY LIST

MONDAY
SNACKS

TUESDAY
SNACKS

WEDNESDAY
SNACKS

THURSDAY
SNACKS

FRIDAY
SNACKS

SATURDAY
SNACKS

SUNDAY
SNACKS

NOTES:

MEAL PLANNER

DATE:

MONDAY
BREAKFAST   LUNCH   DINNER

TUESDAY
BREAKFAST   LUNCH   DINNER

WEDNESDAY
BREAKFAST   LUNCH   DINNER

THURSDAY
BREAKFAST   LUNCH   DINNER

FRIDAY
BREAKFAST   LUNCH   DINNER

SATURDAY
BREAKFAST   LUNCH   DINNER

SUNDAY
BREAKFAST   LUNCH   DINNER

yummy!

MONDAY
SNACKS

TUESDAY
SNACKS

WEDNESDAY
SNACKS

THURSDAY
SNACKS

FRIDAY
SNACKS

SATURDAY
SNACKS

SUNDAY
SNACKS

GROCERY LIST

- _____
- _____
- _____
- _____
- _____
- _____
- _____
- _____
- _____
- _____
- _____
- _____
- _____
- _____
- _____
- _____
- _____
- _____
- _____
- _____
- _____
- _____
- _____

NOTES:

MEAL PLANNER

DATE:

MONDAY
BREAKFAST   LUNCH   DINNER

TUESDAY
BREAKFAST   LUNCH   DINNER

WEDNESDAY
BREAKFAST   LUNCH   DINNER

THURSDAY
BREAKFAST   LUNCH   DINNER

FRIDAY
BREAKFAST   LUNCH   DINNER

SATURDAY
BREAKFAST   LUNCH   DINNER

SUNDAY
BREAKFAST   LUNCH   DINNER

Delicious!

MONDAY — SNACKS

TUESDAY — SNACKS

WEDNESDAY — SNACKS

THURSDAY — SNACKS

FRIDAY — SNACKS

SATURDAY — SNACKS

SUNDAY — SNACKS

GROCERY LIST

- _____
- _____
- _____
- _____
- _____
- _____
- _____
- _____
- _____
- _____
- _____
- _____
- _____
- _____
- _____
- _____
- _____
- _____
- _____
- _____
- _____
- _____
- _____
- _____

NOTES:

MEAL PLANNER

DATE:

	BREAKFAST	LUNCH	DINNER
MONDAY			

	BREAKFAST	LUNCH	DINNER
TUESDAY			

	BREAKFAST	LUNCH	DINNER
WEDNESDAY			

	BREAKFAST	LUNCH	DINNER
THURSDAY			

	BREAKFAST	LUNCH	DINNER
FRIDAY			

	BREAKFAST	LUNCH	DINNER
SATURDAY			

	BREAKFAST	LUNCH	DINNER
SUNDAY			

Tasty!

MONDAY
SNACKS

TUESDAY
SNACKS

WEDNESDAY
SNACKS

THURSDAY
SNACKS

FRIDAY
SNACKS

SATURDAY
SNACKS

SUNDAY
SNACKS

GROCERY LIST

- _____
- _____
- _____
- _____
- _____
- _____
- _____
- _____
- _____
- _____
- _____
- _____
- _____
- _____
- _____
- _____
- _____
- _____
- _____
- _____
- _____
- _____
- _____
- _____
- _____

NOTES:

MEAL PLANNER

DATE:

MONDAY
BREAKFAST   LUNCH   DINNER

TUESDAY
BREAKFAST   LUNCH   DINNER

WEDNESDAY
BREAKFAST   LUNCH   DINNER

THURSDAY
BREAKFAST   LUNCH   DINNER

FRIDAY
BREAKFAST   LUNCH   DINNER

SATURDAY
BREAKFAST   LUNCH   DINNER

SUNDAY
BREAKFAST   LUNCH   DINNER

Scrumptious!

GROCERY LIST

MONDAY

SNACKS

TUESDAY

SNACKS

WEDNESDAY

SNACKS

THURSDAY

SNACKS

FRIDAY

SNACKS

SATURDAY

SNACKS

SUNDAY

SNACKS

NOTES:

MEAL PLANNER

DATE:

MONDAY
BREAKFAST LUNCH DINNER

TUESDAY
BREAKFAST LUNCH DINNER

WEDNESDAY
BREAKFAST LUNCH DINNER

THURSDAY
BREAKFAST LUNCH DINNER

FRIDAY
BREAKFAST LUNCH DINNER

SATURDAY
BREAKFAST LUNCH DINNER

SUNDAY
BREAKFAST LUNCH DINNER

Delectable!

MONDAY
SNACKS

TUESDAY
SNACKS

WEDNESDAY
SNACKS

THURSDAY
SNACKS

FRIDAY
SNACKS

SATURDAY
SNACKS

SUNDAY
SNACKS

NOTES:

MEAL PLANNER

DATE:

MONDAY
BREAKFAST   LUNCH   DINNER

TUESDAY
BREAKFAST   LUNCH   DINNER

WEDNESDAY
BREAKFAST   LUNCH   DINNER

THURSDAY
BREAKFAST   LUNCH   DINNER

FRIDAY
BREAKFAST   LUNCH   DINNER

SATURDAY
BREAKFAST   LUNCH   DINNER

SUNDAY
BREAKFAST   LUNCH   DINNER

yummy!

GROCERY LIST

MONDAY
SNACKS

TUESDAY
SNACKS

WEDNESDAY
SNACKS

THURSDAY
SNACKS

FRIDAY
SNACKS

SATURDAY
SNACKS

SUNDAY
SNACKS

NOTES:

MEAL PLANNER

DATE:

MONDAY
BREAKFAST   LUNCH   DINNER

TUESDAY
BREAKFAST   LUNCH   DINNER

WEDNESDAY
BREAKFAST   LUNCH   DINNER

THURSDAY
BREAKFAST   LUNCH   DINNER

FRIDAY
BREAKFAST   LUNCH   DINNER

SATURDAY
BREAKFAST   LUNCH   DINNER

SUNDAY
BREAKFAST   LUNCH   DINNER

Delicious!

MONDAY
SNACKS

TUESDAY
SNACKS

WEDNESDAY
SNACKS

THURSDAY
SNACKS

FRIDAY
SNACKS

SATURDAY
SNACKS

SUNDAY
SNACKS

GROCERY LIST

- _____
- _____
- _____
- _____
- _____
- _____
- _____
- _____
- _____
- _____
- _____
- _____
- _____
- _____
- _____
- _____
- _____
- _____
- _____
- _____
- _____
- _____
- _____

NOTES:

MEAL PLANNER

DATE:

MONDAY
BREAKFAST | LUNCH | DINNER

TUESDAY
BREAKFAST | LUNCH | DINNER

WEDNESDAY
BREAKFAST | LUNCH | DINNER

THURSDAY
BREAKFAST | LUNCH | DINNER

FRIDAY
BREAKFAST | LUNCH | DINNER

SATURDAY
BREAKFAST | LUNCH | DINNER

SUNDAY
BREAKFAST | LUNCH | DINNER

Tasty!

MONDAY | SNACKS

TUESDAY | SNACKS

WEDNESDAY | SNACKS

THURSDAY | SNACKS

FRIDAY | SNACKS

SATURDAY | SNACKS

SUNDAY | SNACKS

GROCERY LIST

- _____
- _____
- _____
- _____
- _____
- _____
- _____
- _____
- _____
- _____
- _____
- _____
- _____
- _____
- _____
- _____
- _____
- _____
- _____
- _____
- _____
- _____

NOTES:

MEAL PLANNER

DATE:

MONDAY
BREAKFAST | LUNCH | DINNER

TUESDAY
BREAKFAST | LUNCH | DINNER

WEDNESDAY
BREAKFAST | LUNCH | DINNER

THURSDAY
BREAKFAST | LUNCH | DINNER

FRIDAY
BREAKFAST | LUNCH | DINNER

SATURDAY
BREAKFAST | LUNCH | DINNER

SUNDAY
BREAKFAST | LUNCH | DINNER

scrumptious!

GROCERY LIST

MONDAY SNACKS

TUESDAY SNACKS

WEDNESDAY SNACKS

THURSDAY SNACKS

FRIDAY SNACKS

SATURDAY SNACKS

SUNDAY SNACKS

- _____
- _____
- _____
- _____
- _____
- _____
- _____
- _____
- _____
- _____
- _____
- _____
- _____
- _____
- _____
- _____
- _____
- _____
- _____
- _____
- _____
- _____
- _____
- _____
- _____

NOTES:

MEAL PLANNER

DATE:

MONDAY
BREAKFAST	LUNCH	DINNER

TUESDAY
BREAKFAST	LUNCH	DINNER

WEDNESDAY
BREAKFAST	LUNCH	DINNER

THURSDAY
BREAKFAST	LUNCH	DINNER

FRIDAY
BREAKFAST	LUNCH	DINNER

SATURDAY
BREAKFAST	LUNCH	DINNER

SUNDAY
BREAKFAST	LUNCH	DINNER

Delectable!

GROCERY LIST

MONDAY — SNACKS

TUESDAY — SNACKS

WEDNESDAY — SNACKS

THURSDAY — SNACKS

FRIDAY — SNACKS

SATURDAY — SNACKS

SUNDAY — SNACKS

NOTES:

MEAL PLANNER

DATE:

MONDAY	BREAKFAST	LUNCH	DINNER
TUESDAY	BREAKFAST	LUNCH	DINNER
WEDNESDAY	BREAKFAST	LUNCH	DINNER
THURSDAY	BREAKFAST	LUNCH	DINNER
FRIDAY	BREAKFAST	LUNCH	DINNER
SATURDAY	BREAKFAST	LUNCH	DINNER
SUNDAY	BREAKFAST	LUNCH	DINNER

yummy!

MONDAY
SNACKS

TUESDAY
SNACKS

WEDNESDAY
SNACKS

THURSDAY
SNACKS

FRIDAY
SNACKS

SATURDAY
SNACKS

SUNDAY
SNACKS

GROCERY LIST

- _____
- _____
- _____
- _____
- _____
- _____
- _____
- _____
- _____
- _____
- _____
- _____
- _____
- _____
- _____
- _____
- _____
- _____
- _____
- _____
- _____
- _____
- _____

NOTES:

MEAL PLANNER

DATE:

MONDAY
BREAKFAST | LUNCH | DINNER

TUESDAY
BREAKFAST | LUNCH | DINNER

WEDNESDAY
BREAKFAST | LUNCH | DINNER

THURSDAY
BREAKFAST | LUNCH | DINNER

FRIDAY
BREAKFAST | LUNCH | DINNER

SATURDAY
BREAKFAST | LUNCH | DINNER

SUNDAY
BREAKFAST | LUNCH | DINNER

Delicious!

MONDAY
SNACKS

TUESDAY
SNACKS

WEDNESDAY
SNACKS

THURSDAY
SNACKS

FRIDAY
SNACKS

SATURDAY
SNACKS

SUNDAY
SNACKS

GROCERY LIST

- _____
- _____
- _____
- _____
- _____
- _____
- _____
- _____
- _____
- _____
- _____
- _____
- _____
- _____
- _____
- _____
- _____
- _____
- _____
- _____
- _____
- _____
- _____
- _____

NOTES:

MEAL PLANNER

DATE:

MONDAY
BREAKFAST | LUNCH | DINNER

TUESDAY
BREAKFAST | LUNCH | DINNER

WEDNESDAY
BREAKFAST | LUNCH | DINNER

THURSDAY
BREAKFAST | LUNCH | DINNER

FRIDAY
BREAKFAST | LUNCH | DINNER

SATURDAY
BREAKFAST | LUNCH | DINNER

SUNDAY
BREAKFAST | LUNCH | DINNER

Tasty!

MONDAY
SNACKS

TUESDAY
SNACKS

WEDNESDAY
SNACKS

THURSDAY
SNACKS

FRIDAY
SNACKS

SATURDAY
SNACKS

SUNDAY
SNACKS

GROCERY LIST

-
-
-
-
-
-
-
-
-
-
-
-
-
-
-
-
-
-
-
-
-

NOTES:

MEAL PLANNER

DATE:

MONDAY
BREAKFAST LUNCH DINNER

TUESDAY
BREAKFAST LUNCH DINNER

WEDNESDAY
BREAKFAST LUNCH DINNER

THURSDAY
BREAKFAST LUNCH DINNER

FRIDAY
BREAKFAST LUNCH DINNER

SATURDAY
BREAKFAST LUNCH DINNER

SUNDAY
BREAKFAST LUNCH DINNER

scrumptious!

MONDAY
SNACKS

TUESDAY
SNACKS

WEDNESDAY
SNACKS

THURSDAY
SNACKS

FRIDAY
SNACKS

SATURDAY
SNACKS

SUNDAY
SNACKS

GROCERY LIST

- _____
- _____
- _____
- _____
- _____
- _____
- _____
- _____
- _____
- _____
- _____
- _____
- _____
- _____
- _____
- _____
- _____
- _____
- _____
- _____
- _____
- _____
- _____

NOTES:

MEAL PLANNER

DATE:

MONDAY
BREAKFAST LUNCH DINNER

TUESDAY
BREAKFAST LUNCH DINNER

WEDNESDAY
BREAKFAST LUNCH DINNER

THURSDAY
BREAKFAST LUNCH DINNER

FRIDAY
BREAKFAST LUNCH DINNER

SATURDAY
BREAKFAST LUNCH DINNER

SUNDAY
BREAKFAST LUNCH DINNER

Delectable!

GROCERY LIST

MONDAY

SNACKS

TUESDAY

SNACKS

WEDNESDAY

SNACKS

THURSDAY

SNACKS

FRIDAY

SNACKS

SATURDAY

SNACKS

SUNDAY

SNACKS

NOTES:

MEAL PLANNER

DATE:

MONDAY
BREAKFAST　　　　LUNCH　　　　DINNER

TUESDAY
BREAKFAST　　　　LUNCH　　　　DINNER

WEDNESDAY
BREAKFAST　　　　LUNCH　　　　DINNER

THURSDAY
BREAKFAST　　　　LUNCH　　　　DINNER

FRIDAY
BREAKFAST　　　　LUNCH　　　　DINNER

SATURDAY
BREAKFAST　　　　LUNCH　　　　DINNER

SUNDAY
BREAKFAST　　　　LUNCH　　　　DINNER

yummy!

MONDAY
SNACKS

TUESDAY
SNACKS

WEDNESDAY
SNACKS

THURSDAY
SNACKS

FRIDAY
SNACKS

SATURDAY
SNACKS

SUNDAY
SNACKS

GROCERY LIST

- _____
- _____
- _____
- _____
- _____
- _____
- _____
- _____
- _____
- _____
- _____
- _____
- _____
- _____
- _____
- _____
- _____
- _____
- _____
- _____
- _____
- _____

NOTES:

MEAL PLANNER

DATE:

MONDAY
BREAKFAST   LUNCH   DINNER

TUESDAY
BREAKFAST   LUNCH   DINNER

WEDNESDAY
BREAKFAST   LUNCH   DINNER

THURSDAY
BREAKFAST   LUNCH   DINNER

FRIDAY
BREAKFAST   LUNCH   DINNER

SATURDAY
BREAKFAST   LUNCH   DINNER

SUNDAY
BREAKFAST   LUNCH   DINNER

Delicious!

GROCERY LIST

MONDAY — SNACKS

TUESDAY — SNACKS

WEDNESDAY — SNACKS

THURSDAY — SNACKS

FRIDAY — SNACKS

SATURDAY — SNACKS

SUNDAY — SNACKS

NOTES:

MEAL PLANNER

DATE:

	BREAKFAST	LUNCH	DINNER
MONDAY			

	BREAKFAST	LUNCH	DINNER
TUESDAY			

	BREAKFAST	LUNCH	DINNER
WEDNESDAY			

	BREAKFAST	LUNCH	DINNER
THURSDAY			

	BREAKFAST	LUNCH	DINNER
FRIDAY			

	BREAKFAST	LUNCH	DINNER
SATURDAY			

	BREAKFAST	LUNCH	DINNER
SUNDAY			

Tasty!

GROCERY LIST

MONDAY
SNACKS

TUESDAY
SNACKS

WEDNESDAY
SNACKS

THURSDAY
SNACKS

FRIDAY
SNACKS

SATURDAY
SNACKS

SUNDAY
SNACKS

NOTES:

MEAL PLANNER

DATE:

MONDAY	BREAKFAST	LUNCH	DINNER

TUESDAY	BREAKFAST	LUNCH	DINNER

WEDNESDAY	BREAKFAST	LUNCH	DINNER

THURSDAY	BREAKFAST	LUNCH	DINNER

FRIDAY	BREAKFAST	LUNCH	DINNER

SATURDAY	BREAKFAST	LUNCH	DINNER

SUNDAY	BREAKFAST	LUNCH	DINNER

scrumptious!

GROCERY LIST

MONDAY
SNACKS

TUESDAY
SNACKS

WEDNESDAY
SNACKS

THURSDAY
SNACKS

FRIDAY
SNACKS

SATURDAY
SNACKS

SUNDAY
SNACKS

NOTES:

MEAL PLANNER

DATE:

MONDAY	BREAKFAST	LUNCH	DINNER

TUESDAY	BREAKFAST	LUNCH	DINNER

WEDNESDAY	BREAKFAST	LUNCH	DINNER

THURSDAY	BREAKFAST	LUNCH	DINNER

FRIDAY	BREAKFAST	LUNCH	DINNER

SATURDAY	BREAKFAST	LUNCH	DINNER

SUNDAY	BREAKFAST	LUNCH	DINNER

Delectable!

GROCERY LIST

MONDAY
SNACKS

TUESDAY
SNACKS

WEDNESDAY
SNACKS

THURSDAY
SNACKS

FRIDAY
SNACKS

SATURDAY
SNACKS

SUNDAY
SNACKS

NOTES:

MEAL PLANNER

DATE:

MONDAY
BREAKFAST   LUNCH   DINNER

TUESDAY
BREAKFAST   LUNCH   DINNER

WEDNESDAY
BREAKFAST   LUNCH   DINNER

THURSDAY
BREAKFAST   LUNCH   DINNER

FRIDAY
BREAKFAST   LUNCH   DINNER

SATURDAY
BREAKFAST   LUNCH   DINNER

SUNDAY
BREAKFAST   LUNCH   DINNER

yummy!

GROCERY LIST

MONDAY — SNACKS

TUESDAY — SNACKS

WEDNESDAY — SNACKS

THURSDAY — SNACKS

FRIDAY — SNACKS

SATURDAY — SNACKS

SUNDAY — SNACKS

NOTES:

MEAL PLANNER

DATE:

MONDAY
BREAKFAST	LUNCH	DINNER

TUESDAY
BREAKFAST	LUNCH	DINNER

WEDNESDAY
BREAKFAST	LUNCH	DINNER

THURSDAY
BREAKFAST	LUNCH	DINNER

FRIDAY
BREAKFAST	LUNCH	DINNER

SATURDAY
BREAKFAST	LUNCH	DINNER

SUNDAY
BREAKFAST	LUNCH	DINNER

Delicious!

GROCERY LIST

MONDAY · SNACKS

TUESDAY · SNACKS

WEDNESDAY · SNACKS

THURSDAY · SNACKS

FRIDAY · SNACKS

SATURDAY · SNACKS

SUNDAY · SNACKS

NOTES:

MEAL PLANNER

DATE:

| MONDAY | BREAKFAST | LUNCH | DINNER |

| TUESDAY | BREAKFAST | LUNCH | DINNER |

| WEDNESDAY | BREAKFAST | LUNCH | DINNER |

| THURSDAY | BREAKFAST | LUNCH | DINNER |

| FRIDAY | BREAKFAST | LUNCH | DINNER |

| SATURDAY | BREAKFAST | LUNCH | DINNER |

| SUNDAY | BREAKFAST | LUNCH | DINNER |

Tasty!

MONDAY
SNACKS

TUESDAY
SNACKS

WEDNESDAY
SNACKS

THURSDAY
SNACKS

FRIDAY
SNACKS

SATURDAY
SNACKS

SUNDAY
SNACKS

GROCERY LIST

- _____
- _____
- _____
- _____
- _____
- _____
- _____
- _____
- _____
- _____
- _____
- _____
- _____
- _____
- _____
- _____
- _____
- _____
- _____
- _____
- _____
- _____

NOTES:

MEAL PLANNER

DATE:

MONDAY
BREAKFAST	LUNCH	DINNER

TUESDAY
BREAKFAST	LUNCH	DINNER

WEDNESDAY
BREAKFAST	LUNCH	DINNER

THURSDAY
BREAKFAST	LUNCH	DINNER

FRIDAY
BREAKFAST	LUNCH	DINNER

SATURDAY
BREAKFAST	LUNCH	DINNER

SUNDAY
BREAKFAST	LUNCH	DINNER

scrumptious!

GROCERY LIST

MONDAY — SNACKS

TUESDAY — SNACKS

WEDNESDAY — SNACKS

THURSDAY — SNACKS

FRIDAY — SNACKS

SATURDAY — SNACKS

SUNDAY — SNACKS

NOTES:

MEAL PLANNER

DATE:

MONDAY
BREAKFAST | LUNCH | DINNER

TUESDAY
BREAKFAST | LUNCH | DINNER

WEDNESDAY
BREAKFAST | LUNCH | DINNER

THURSDAY
BREAKFAST | LUNCH | DINNER

FRIDAY
BREAKFAST | LUNCH | DINNER

SATURDAY
BREAKFAST | LUNCH | DINNER

SUNDAY
BREAKFAST | LUNCH | DINNER

Delectable!

MONDAY
SNACKS

TUESDAY
SNACKS

WEDNESDAY
SNACKS

THURSDAY
SNACKS

FRIDAY
SNACKS

SATURDAY
SNACKS

SUNDAY
SNACKS

GROCERY LIST

- _____
- _____
- _____
- _____
- _____
- _____
- _____
- _____
- _____
- _____
- _____
- _____
- _____
- _____
- _____
- _____
- _____
- _____
- _____
- _____
- _____
- _____
- _____

NOTES:

MEAL PLANNER

DATE:

MONDAY	BREAKFAST	LUNCH	DINNER

TUESDAY	BREAKFAST	LUNCH	DINNER

WEDNESDAY	BREAKFAST	LUNCH	DINNER

THURSDAY	BREAKFAST	LUNCH	DINNER

FRIDAY	BREAKFAST	LUNCH	DINNER

SATURDAY	BREAKFAST	LUNCH	DINNER

SUNDAY	BREAKFAST	LUNCH	DINNER

yummy!

GROCERY LIST

MONDAY — SNACKS

TUESDAY — SNACKS

WEDNESDAY — SNACKS

THURSDAY — SNACKS

FRIDAY — SNACKS

SATURDAY — SNACKS

SUNDAY — SNACKS

NOTES:

MEAL PLANNER

DATE:

MONDAY
BREAKFAST   LUNCH   DINNER

TUESDAY
BREAKFAST   LUNCH   DINNER

WEDNESDAY
BREAKFAST   LUNCH   DINNER

THURSDAY
BREAKFAST   LUNCH   DINNER

FRIDAY
BREAKFAST   LUNCH   DINNER

SATURDAY
BREAKFAST   LUNCH   DINNER

SUNDAY
BREAKFAST   LUNCH   DINNER

Delicious!

MONDAY
SNACKS

TUESDAY
SNACKS

WEDNESDAY
SNACKS

THURSDAY
SNACKS

FRIDAY
SNACKS

SATURDAY
SNACKS

SUNDAY
SNACKS

GROCERY LIST

- _____
- _____
- _____
- _____
- _____
- _____
- _____
- _____
- _____
- _____
- _____
- _____
- _____
- _____
- _____
- _____
- _____
- _____
- _____
- _____
- _____
- _____
- _____
- _____

NOTES:

MEAL PLANNER

DATE:

MONDAY | BREAKFAST | LUNCH | DINNER

TUESDAY | BREAKFAST | LUNCH | DINNER

WEDNESDAY | BREAKFAST | LUNCH | DINNER

THURSDAY | BREAKFAST | LUNCH | DINNER

FRIDAY | BREAKFAST | LUNCH | DINNER

SATURDAY | BREAKFAST | LUNCH | DINNER

SUNDAY | BREAKFAST | LUNCH | DINNER

Tasty!

MONDAY
SNACKS

TUESDAY
SNACKS

WEDNESDAY
SNACKS

THURSDAY
SNACKS

FRIDAY
SNACKS

SATURDAY
SNACKS

SUNDAY
SNACKS

GROCERY LIST

NOTES:

THANK YOU SO MUCH

FOR PURCHASING OUR BOOK.

WE HOPE YOU HAVE FOUND THIS PLANNER

HELPFUL AND FUN.

PLEASE LEAVE AN HONEST REVIEW!

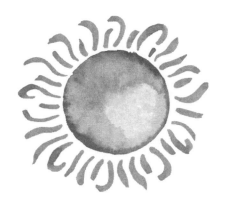

TO SEE ALL OUR LATEST BOOKS OR LEAVE A REVIEW

PLEASE GO TO

sunnymorningbooks.com

YOUR SUPPORT IS MUCH APPRECIATED.